Keto Diet Cookbook for Vegetarians

Easy and Tasty Recipes for Vegetarians on a Ketogenic Diet

By

Elisa Hayes

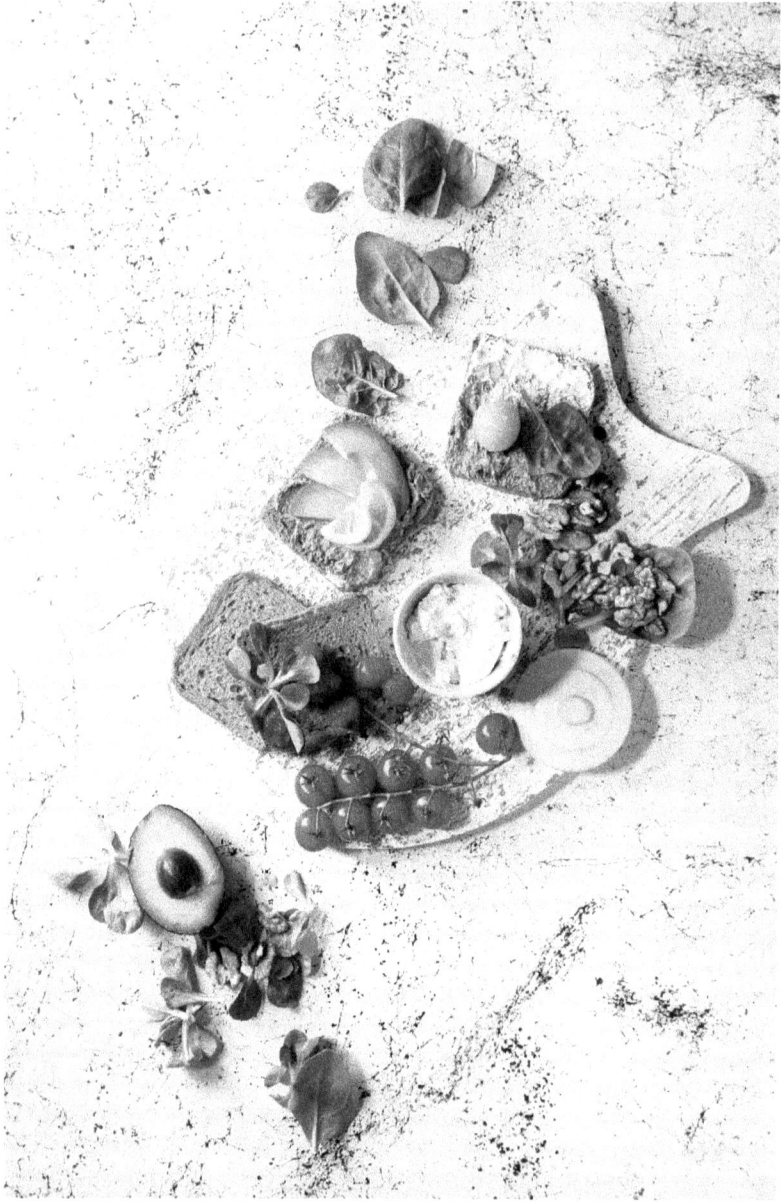

Table of Contents

Furthermore, the transmission, duplication, or reproduction of any of the following work including specific information will be considered an illegal act irrespective of if it is done electronically or in print. This extends to creating a secondary or tertiary copy of the work or a recorded copy and is only allowed with the express written consent from the Publisher. All additional rights reserved.

The information in the following pages is broadly considered a truthful and accurate account of facts and as such, any inattention, use, or misuse of the information in question by the reader will render any resulting actions solely under their purview. There are no scenarios in which the publisher or the original author of this work can be in any fashion deemed liable for any hardship or damages that may befall them after undertaking information described herein.

Additionally, the information in the following pages is intended only for informational purposes and should thus be thought of as universal. As befitting its nature, it is presented without assurance regarding its prolonged validity or interim quality. Trademarks that are mentioned are done without written consent and can in no way be considered an endorsement from the trademark holder.

Introduction

The path to a perfect body and good physical health was very thorny for me. The only one wish which I was making for my birthdays for many years was to be a slim and beautiful girl. Alas, everything can't be as in fairy tales and the miracle didn't happen; my mirror was still showing the same fat, pimple girl. In childhood, the problem of being overweight didn't bother me much; I can say that I didn't care about it at all, I didn't know that weight would be momentous for me. I was an ordinary smiling child, playing with my peers, going to school, and traveling with my parents. That time my chubby cheeks seemed very sweet to everyone. But that was then. At 11-year-old, I went to middle school. New people, new teachers, I had no friends at all. Mentally I was broken. I counted the minutes until the end of the last lesson, to quickly sit in my mom's car and leave school. I started to eat a lot. Now I see that in this way I am stressed, but then the food served as my antidepressant. Dozens of hamburgers, fried potatoes, coke – they were "my best friends". In addition to everything, I started to have horrible skin problems, it seemed to me that there was no place on my face wherever they hadn't appeared yet. Time passed and I no longer loved my reflection in the mirror even in 1%. I couldn't wear the clothes that I liked. I usually wore oversized shorts and t-shirts. I couldn't afford to wear a short dress and high heels. At 15-year-old I weighed more than 270lbs. I remember what I felt in those days, as it is happening now. I felt anger, irritation, hatred, and self-loathing. That prom party was the most terrible day of my life. Thank God it's over!

In those years, the keto diet was not very popular, fasting and drinking diets (which, as you already know, did not help me much) were more popular. Perhaps I wouldn't do anything, but my health problems were becoming more serious. It seemed that my body was simply screaming: please help me!

I remember the day that changed my life on a dime. I came to the clinic with pain in my stomach. But this time, I not only received painkillers but also found a mentor and friend. This was my physician. She had examined me and recommended that I go on a diet. I didn't want to do something and was categorically against it. However, my mind changed when she said: love your body, care about it, and it will thank you. What was my surprise when the diet turned out to be very simple to follow. Is it so easy to love myself? As you could understand I am talking about my favorite keto diet. Every day I was eating a maximum of proteins and a minimum of carbohydrates. That meant to consume meat, poultry, and fish and make restrictions for vegetables, fruits, and sweets. After 2 weeks, I lost 83lbs, and further results were getting better and better. All this time I was under the supervision of a doctor and this yielded results. A year later, I completely changed all the clothes in my wardrobe and oh my God I was able to wear a short dress and skirts! Now I can say that I am the happiest person. It happened because I fell in love with myself and started treating my body as a diamond. My life was filled with bright colors, I have a beloved husband, children, work, friends, I am healthy and like myself in the mirror. I am telling this story to prove that the right diet can solve almost all problems with body and health. It is a fact that our body is capable of dealing with dramatic changes, it is only worth loving it. Never rest on your laurels, never give up and forbid people to say that you cannot do something. You are already a great fellow that you bought this cookbook and decided to take a step ahead in the direction to your dream. Let this book become your ray of hope, a lifesaver on the way to your wonderful transformation. If you believe in yourself and love your body, believe me, the result won't be long in coming. You will see in the mirror a completely new version of yourself, updated physically and mentally! Just trust the keto diet and your inner voice. Set a goal today and start the way of achieving it right now. Don't try to do it all in one time; let it be a small step day by day. Exactly now, this is the right time to start creating a new version of you. If this diet was able to change my life, I'm sure it will help you too!

Bacon Broccoli Mash

Prep time: 10 minutes

Cook time: 0 minutes

Servings: 5

Ingredients:

- 2-pounds broccoli, boiled
- 2 oz bacon, chopped, roasted
- ¼ cup coconut cream
- 1 teaspoon salt

Method:

1. Put the cooked broccoli in the food processor.

2. Add coconut cream and salt. Blend the mixture until smooth.

3. Then add bacon and mix the cooked mash.

Nutritional info per serve: Calories 134, Fat 7.8, Fiber 4.8, Carbs 10.4, Protein 8.1

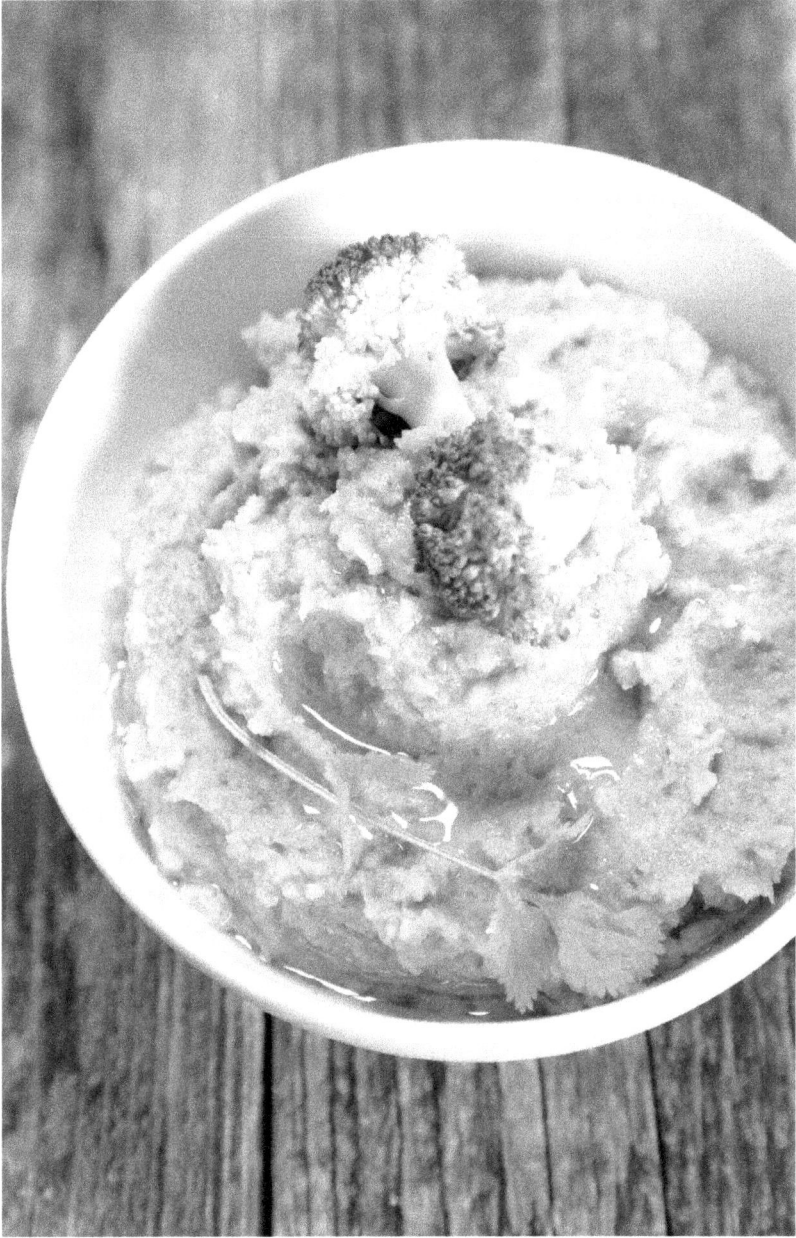

Parsley Asparagus

Prep time: 10 minutes

Cook time: 20 minutes

Servings:4

Ingredients:

- 1-pound asparagus
- 1 teaspoon dried parsley
- ½ teaspoon salt
- 1 tablespoon coconut oil

Method:

1. Mix the asparagus with dried parsley and salt.

2. Put the vegetables in the baking tray. Add coconut oil.

3. Cook the asparagus in the oven at 360F for 20 minutes.

Nutritional info per serve: Calories 52, Fat 3.5, Fiber 2.4, Carbs 4.4, Protein 2.5

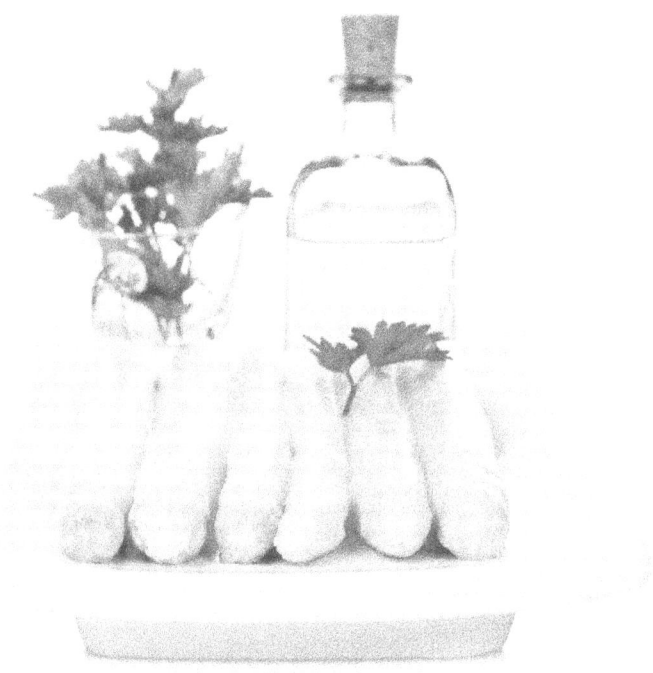

Marinated Broccoli

Prep time: 10 minutes

Cook time: 20 minutes

Servings: 4

Ingredients:

- 2 cups broccoli, chopped, boiled
- 3 tablespoons apple cider vinegar
- 1 teaspoon chili flakes
- 1 tablespoon olive oil
- ½ teaspoon salt

Method:

1. Mix the broccoli with apple cider vinegar, chili flakes, and olive oil.

2. Add salt and mix the broccoli well. Leave it in the fridge for 20 minutes to marinate.

Nutritional info per serve: Calories 48, Fat 3.7, Fiber 1.2, Carbs 3.1, Protein 1.3

Lemon Bell Peppers

Prep time: 10 minutes

Cook time: 8 minutes

Servings:2

Ingredients:

- 1 cup bell pepper, trimmed
- 1 teaspoon minced garlic
- 1 tablespoon avocado oil
- 1 tablespoon lemon juice

Method:

1. Pierce the bell peppers with the help of the knife and put in the hot skillet.

2. Roast the bell peppers for 4 minutes per side.

3. After this, peel the peppers and slice them.

4. Add avocado oil, lemon juice, and minced garlic. Mix the bell peppers.

Nutritional info per serve: Calories 32, Fat 1.1, Fiber 1.2, Carbs 5.5, Protein 0.8

Watercress Soup

Prep time: 10 minutes

Cook time: 15 minutes

Servings: 4

Ingredients:

- 2 spring onions, chopped
- 6 oz watercress, chopped
- 4 cups chicken broth
- 1 teaspoon ground black pepper
- 1 teaspoon olive oil

Method:

1. Roast the spring onion with olive oil in the saucepan for 2 minutes per side.

2. Add watercress, chicken broth, ground black pepper, and close the lid.

3. Simmer the soup for 10 minutes on medium heat.

Nutritional info per serve: Calories 69, Fat 2.8, Fiber 1.2, Carbs 4, Protein 6.4

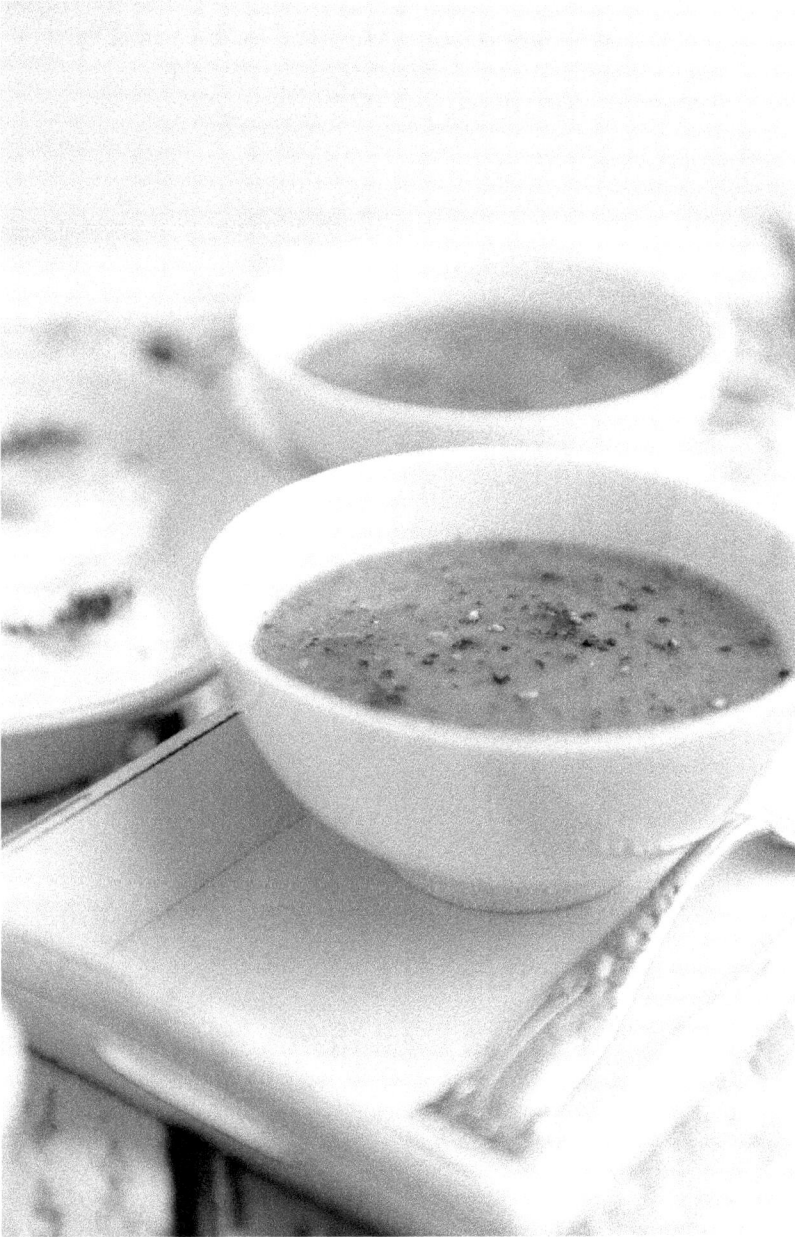

Garlic Cauliflower Fritters

Prep time: 15 minutes

Cook time: 10 minutes

Servings:5

Ingredients:

- 1 cup cauliflower, shredded
- 1 egg, beaten
- 1 oz Cheddar cheese, shredded
- 1 teaspoon minced garlic
- 2 tablespoons almond flour
- 1 tablespoon coconut oil

Method:

1. Mix shredded cauliflower with egg, cheese, minced garlic, and almond flour.

2. Make the fritters and roast them in the hot coconut oil for 5 minutes per side.

Nutritional info per serve: Calories 129, Fat 11.1, Fiber 1.7, Carbs 3.8, Protein 5.4

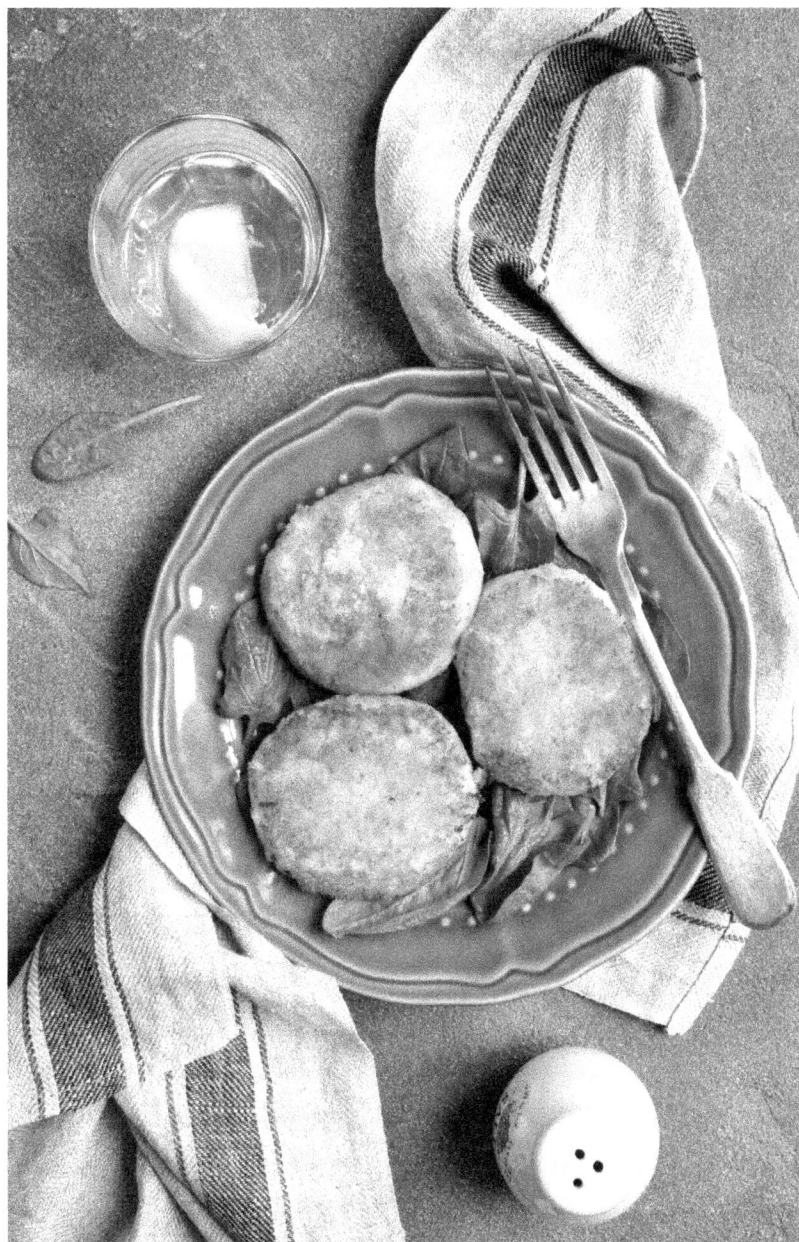

Coconut Mushroom Cream Soup

Prep time: 10 minutes

Cook time: 25 minutes

Servings: 4

Ingredients:

- 3 oz Parmesan, grated
- 1 cup of coconut milk
- 3 cups of water
- 2 scallions, diced
- 1 tablespoon avocado oil
- 2 cups mushrooms, chopped

Method:

1. Pour the avocado oil in the saucepan and preheat.

2. Add mushrooms and scallions. Roast the vegetables for 10 minutes on the medium heat.

3. After this, add water, coconut milk, and Parmesan. Stir the soup and bring to boil.

4. Simmer the soup for 10 minutes. Then blend it until smooth with the help of the immersion blender.

Nutritional info per serve: Calories 161, Fat 13.9, Fiber 2.1, Carbs 4.7, Protein 6.7

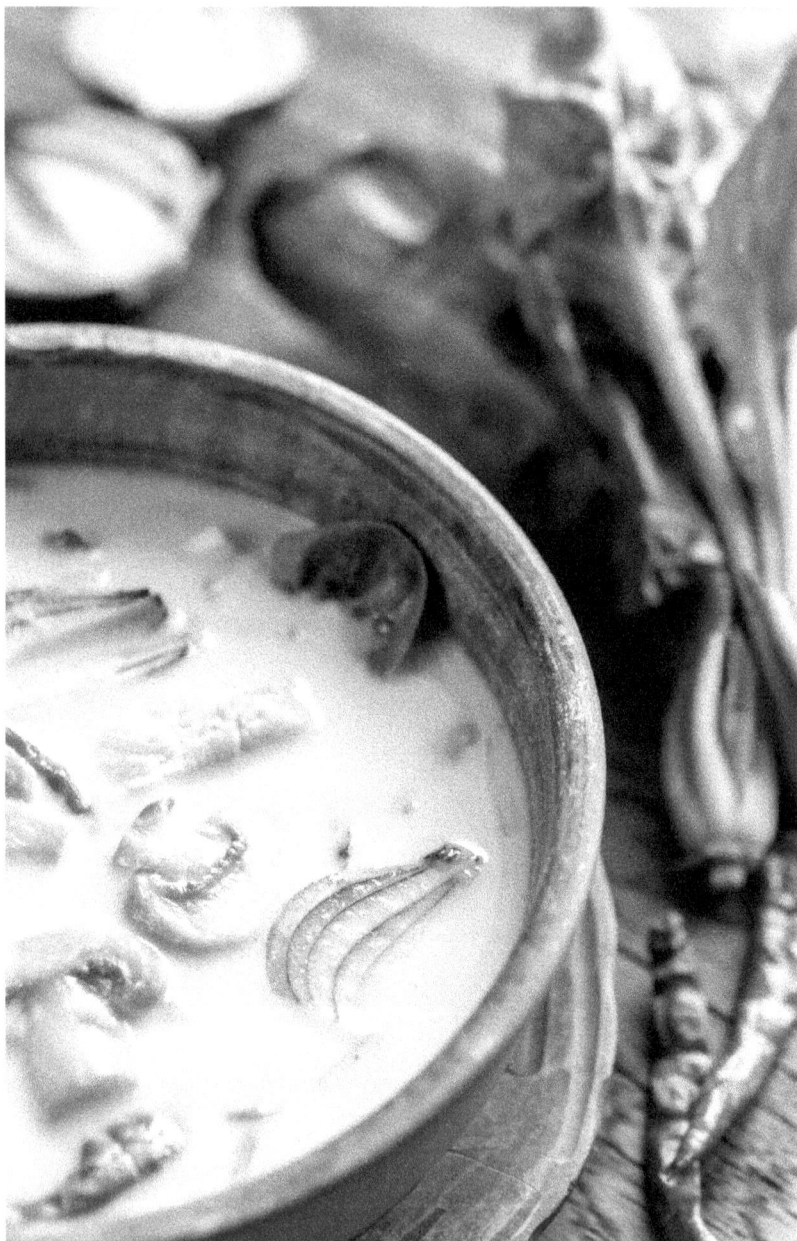

Rosemary Grilled Peppers

Prep time: 10 minutes

Cook time: 5 minutes

Servings: 4

Ingredients:

- 1 cup bell peppers, roughly chopped
- 1 teaspoon dried rosemary
- 1 tablespoon avocado oil
- ½ teaspoon salt

Method:

1. Mix the bell peppers with dried rosemary, avocado oil, and salt.

2. Then preheat the grill to 400F.

3. Put the bell peppers in the frill and roast them for 2 minutes per side.

Nutritional info per serve: Calories 15, Fat 0.6, Fiber 0.7, Carbs 2.6, Protein 0.4

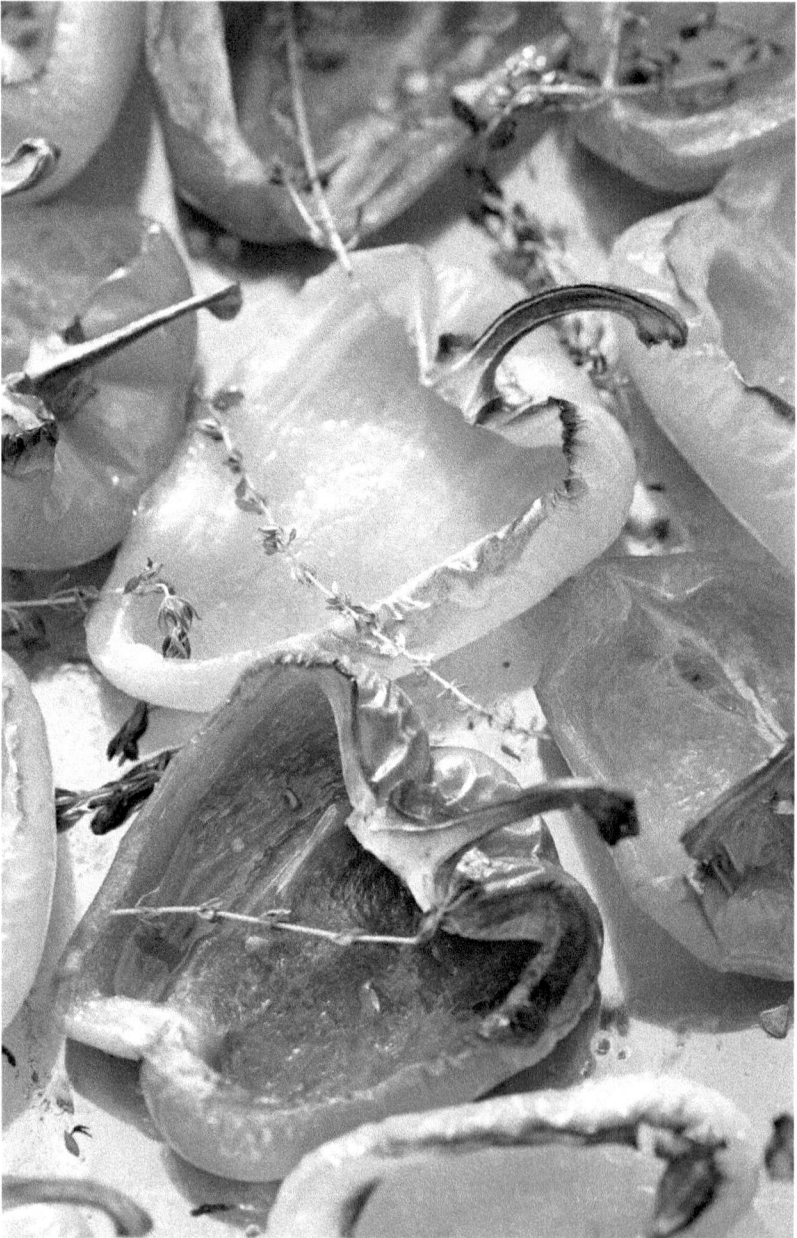

Roasted Bok Choy

Prep time: 10 minutes

Cook time: 10 minutes

Servings: 2

Ingredients:

- 10 oz bok choy, roughly sliced
- 2 oz pancetta, chopped
- 1 teaspoon coconut oil
- ½ teaspoon dried thyme

Method:

1. Put the pancetta in the skillet and roast it for 2 minutes per side.

2. Add coconut oil and melt it.

3. Then add bok choy and dried thyme. Roast the vegetables for 1 minute per side.

Nutritional info per serve: Calories 192, Fat 14.4, Fiber 1.5, Carbs 3.7, Protein 12.7

Baked Rutabaga

Prep time: 10 minutes

Cook time: 10 minutes

Servings:4

Ingredients:

- 2 cups rutabaga, chopped
- 1 tablespoon coconut oil
- 1 teaspoon ground coriander
- ½ teaspoon salt

Method:

1. Mix rutabaga with coconut oil, ground coriander, and salt.

2. Put the vegetables in the baking pan and bake them in the preheated to 360F oven for 10 minutes.

Nutritional info per serve: Calories 55, Fat 3.5, Fiber 1.8, Carbs 5.7, Protein 0.8

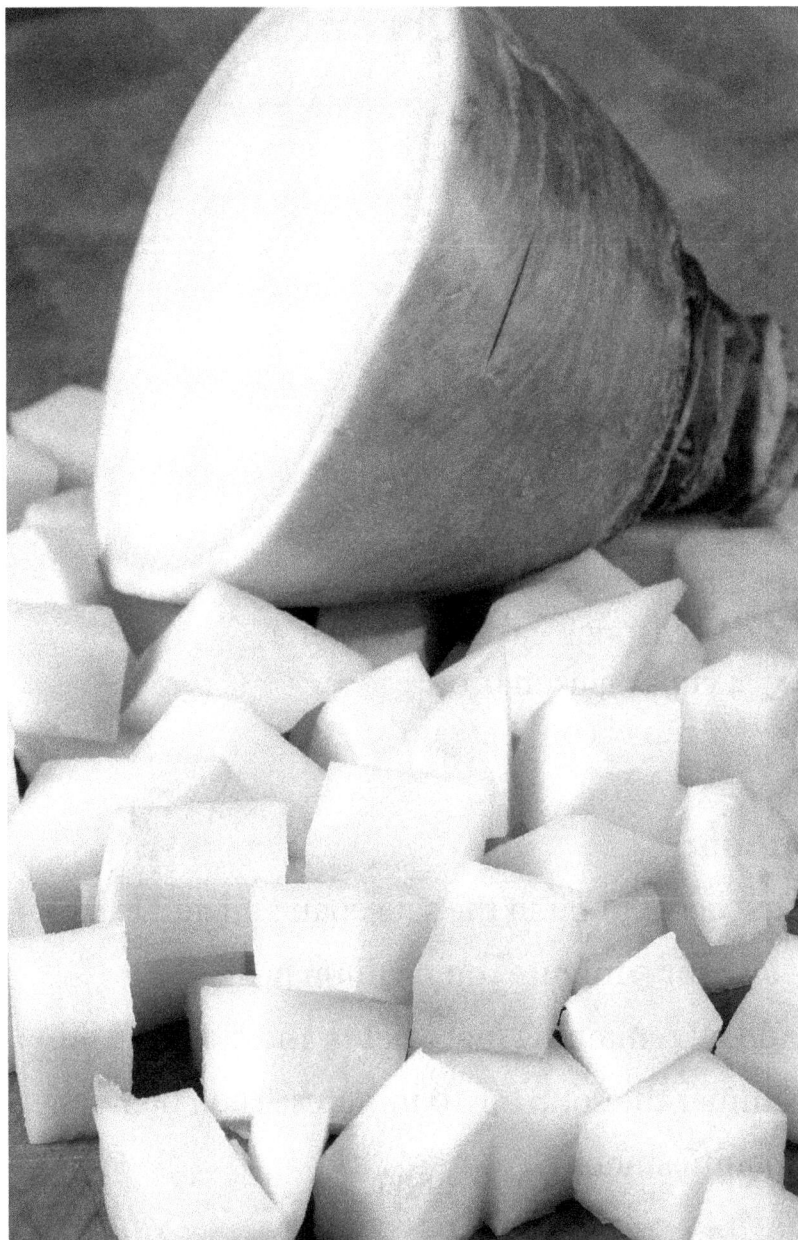

Celery Cream Soup

Prep time: 10 minutes

Cook time: 20 minutes

Servings: 4

Ingredients:

- 1 cup celery stalk, chopped
- ½ cup leek, chopped
- 2 tablespoons coconut oil
- ½ teaspoon cayenne pepper
- 4 cups chicken broth
- ¼ cup coconut cream

Method:

1. Melt coconut oil in the saucepan and add leek. Roast the leek for 5 minutes on medium heat.

2. Add all remaining ingredients and close the lid.

3. Simmer the soup for 10 minutes. Then blend the soup until smooth.

Nutritional info per serve: Calories 143, Fat 11.9, Fiber 1, Carbs 4.2, Protein 5.6

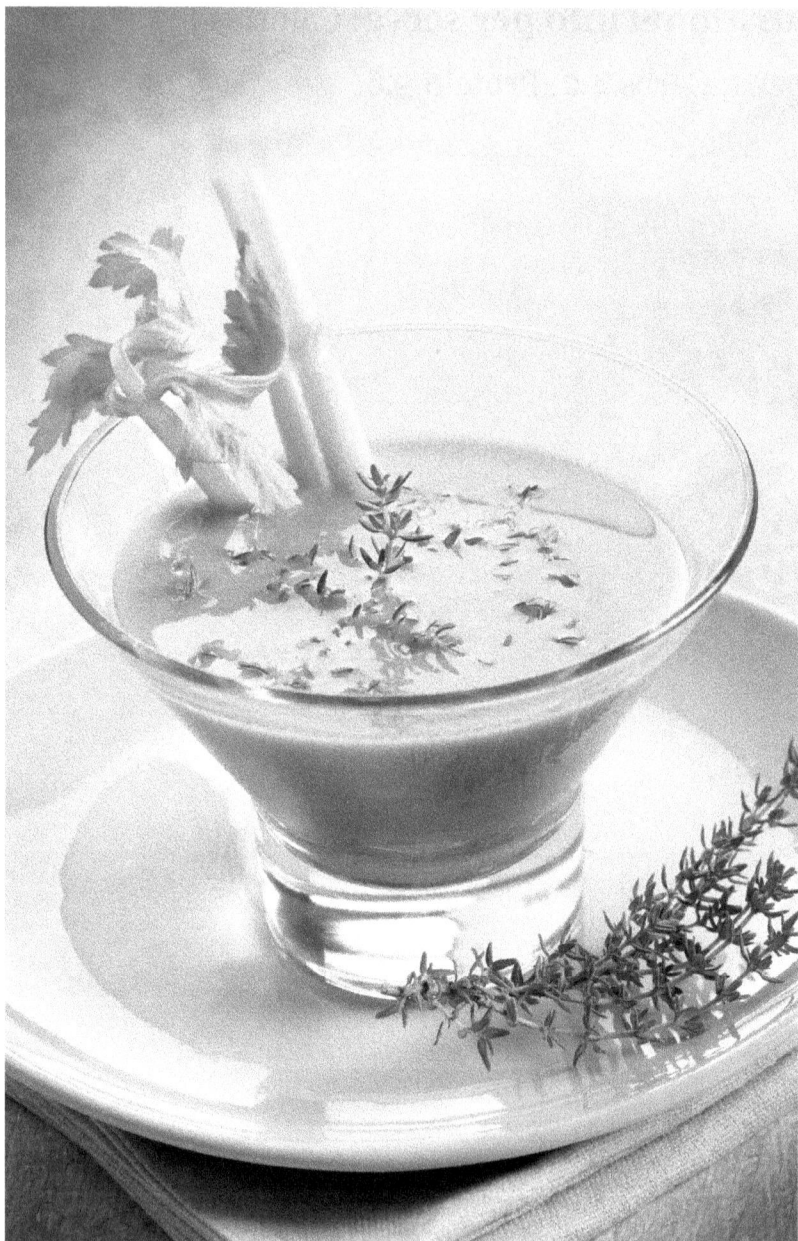

Lettuce Sandwich

Prep time: 10 minutes

Cook time: 0 minutes

Servings: 2

Ingredients:

- 4 lettuce leaves
- 2 Cheddar cheese slices
- 2 teaspoons cream cheese
- 1 teaspoon chives, chopped

Method:

1. Mix cream cheese with chives.

2. Put the chives mixture in 2 lettuce leaves.

3. Add Cheddar cheese slices.

4. Cover the cheese with the remaining lettuce.

Nutritional info per serve: Calories 126, Fat 10.5, Fiber 0.1, Carbs 0.8, Protein 7.3

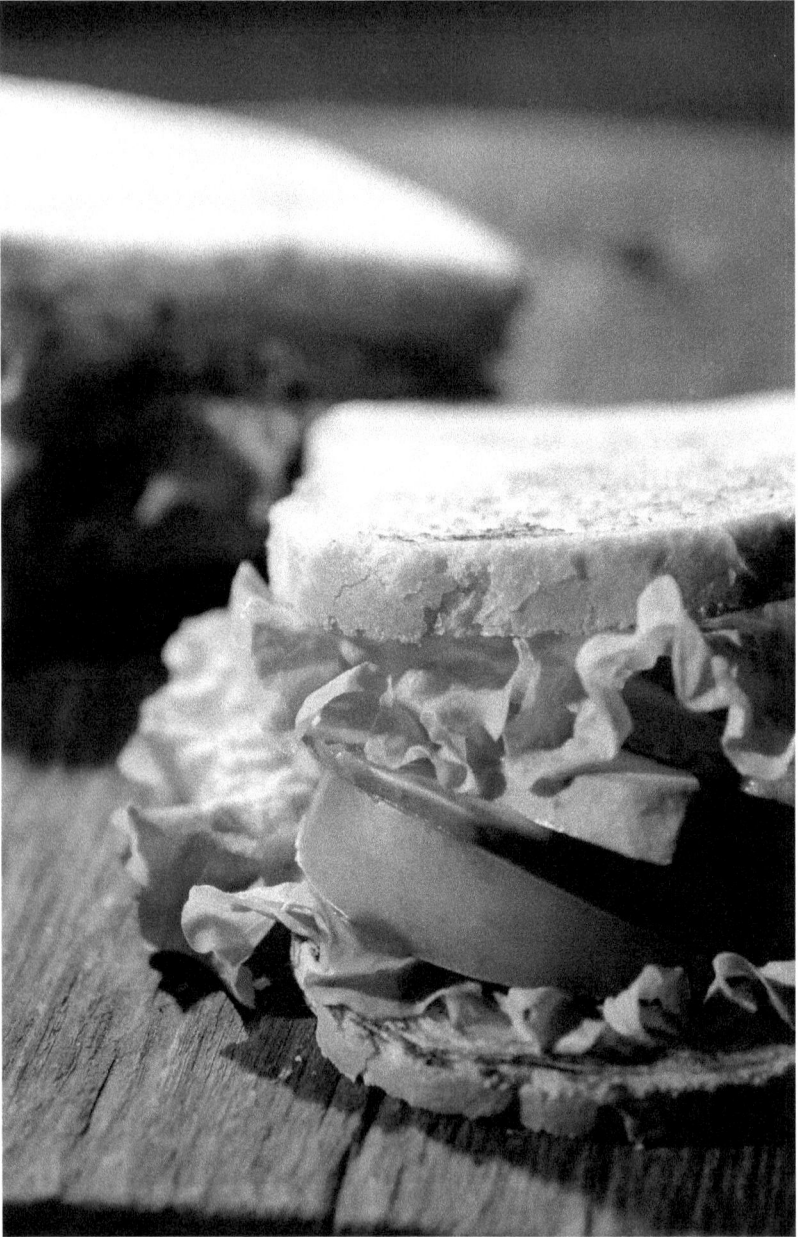

Fenugreek Celery Stalks

Prep time: 10 minutes

Cook time: 5 minutes

Servings: 8

Ingredients:

- 8 celery stalks
- 1 teaspoon fenugreek powder
- 1 tablespoon butter
- ½ teaspoon salt

Method:

1. Melt the butter in the skillet.

2. Add celery stalks and roast them for 1 minute per side.

3. Then sprinkle the celery stalks with salt and fenugreek powder.

4. Roast the vegetables for 2 minutes more.

Nutritional info per serve: Calories 15, Fat 1.5, Fiber 0.3, Carbs 0.5, Protein 0.1

Cauliflower Cream

Prep time: 10 minutes

Cook time: 15 minutes

Servings:4

Ingredients:

- 1 cup organic almond milk
- 1 teaspoon salt
- ¼ cup provolone cheese, shredded
- ½ teaspoon chili powder
- 1 cup cauliflower, chopped
- 1 spring onion, diced
- 1 teaspoon coconut oil

Method:

1. Mix cauliflower with almond milk and boil the mixture for 10 minutes.

2. Then add salt, provolone cheese, chili powder, spring onion, and coconut oil. Simmer the meal for 5 minutes more.

3. Blend the cooked meal until smooth.

Nutritional info per serve: Calories 61, Fat 4.2, Fiber 1, Carbs 3, Protein 3.1

Broccoli Spread

Prep time: 15 minutes

Cook time: 0 minutes

Servings:6

Ingredients:

- 2 cups broccoli, boiled
- 1 oz macadamia nuts, grinded
- 2 tablespoons cream cheese
- ½ teaspoon ground paprika
- ½ cup Cheddar cheese, shredded

Method:

1. Mash the broccoli with the help of the potato masher until smooth.

2. Then add macadamia nuts, cream cheese, ground paprika, and Cheddar cheese.

3. Carefully mix the broccoli spread.

Nutritional info per serve: Calories 94, Fat 8, Fiber 1.3, Carbs 3, Protein 3.9

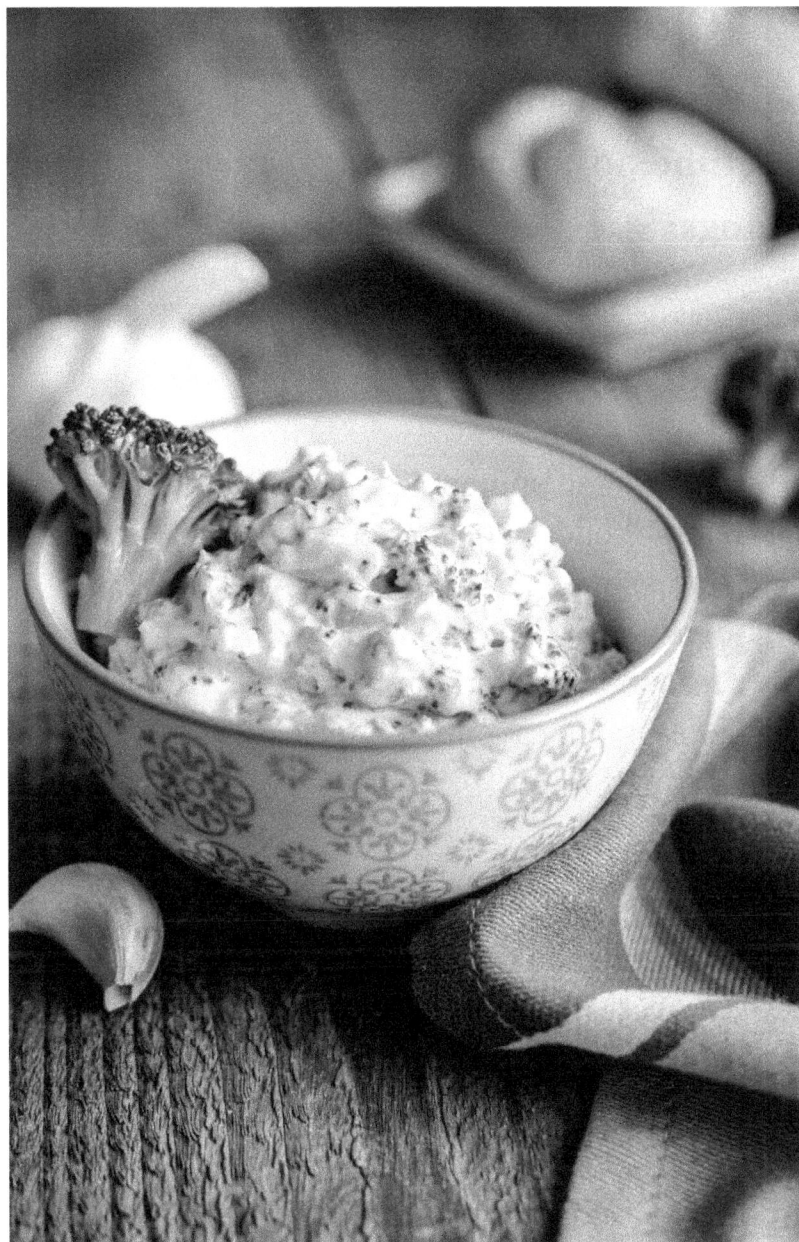

Cheese and Spinach Cream

Prep time: 10 minutes

Cook time: 10 minutes

Servings: 8

Ingredients:

- 3 cups fresh spinach, chopped
- 1 cup Cheddar cheese, shredded
- 2 tablespoons butter
- 1 teaspoon coconut shred
- 1 teaspoon ground paprika
- ½ teaspoon cayenne pepper
- ¼ cup of water

Method:

1. Melt the butter in the saucepan and add spinach. Roast it for 2 minutes.

2. Then stir it and add coconut shred, ground paprika, and cayenne pepper.

3. Add water and simmer the spinach for 5 minutes.

4. Add cheese and carefully mix the cooked meal.

Nutritional info per serve: Calories 88, Fat 7.9, Fiber 0.4, Carbs 0.9, Protein 3.9

Brussel Sprouts Fritters

Prep time: 10 minutes

Cook time: 10 minutes

Servings:6

Ingredients:

- 1 cup Brussel Sprouts, shredded
- 2 eggs, beaten
- 2 tablespoons coconut flour
- 1 teaspoon ground turmeric
- 1 teaspoon ground black pepper
- 1 oz Parmesan, grated
- 1 tablespoon coconut oil

Method:

1. Mix Brussel sprouts with eggs, coconut flour, ground turmeric, ground black pepper, and Parmesan.

2. Make the fritters from the vegetable mixture.

3. Then melt the coconut oil in the skillet.

4. Add fritters and roast them for 4 minutes per side on the medium heat.

Nutritional info per serve: Calories 74, Fat 5.2, Fiber 1.6, Carbs 3.4, Protein 4.3

Lemon Greens

Prep time: 7 minutes

Cook time: 10 minutes

Servings: 4

Ingredients:

- 1 cup collard greens, chopped
- 1 tablespoon butter
- 1 teaspoon lemon zest, grated
- 1 tablespoon lemon juice
- ½ teaspoon smoked paprika

Method:

1. Melt the butter in the skillet.

2. Add all remaining ingredients and mix.

3. Cook the greens on medium heat for 5 minutes.

Nutritional info per serve: Calories 31, Fat 3, Fiber 0.5, Carbs 0.9, Protein 0.4

Garlic Mash

Prep time: 10 minutes

Cook time: 0 minutes

Servings:3

Ingredients:

- 1 cup cauliflower, boiled, mashed
- 1 teaspoon minced garlic
- 2 tablespoons butter
- ¼ cup of coconut milk

Method:

1. Put all ingredients in the mixing bowl.
2. Carefully mix the garlic mash.

Nutritional info per serve: Calories 124, Fat 12.5, Fiber 1.3, Carbs 3.2, Protein 1.3

Buttered Onion

Prep time: 5 minutes

Cook time: 10 minutes

Servings: 4

Ingredients:

- 3 spring onions, sliced
- 3 tablespoons butter
- ½ teaspoon Erythritol

Method:

1. Melt the butter in the skillet.

2. Add spring onion and cook it for 4 minutes on medium heat.

3. Then add Erythritol and carefully mix the onion.

4. Cook it on low heat for 5 minutes more.

Nutritional info per serve: Calories 87, Fat 8.7, Fiber 0.6, Carbs 2.6, Protein 0.4

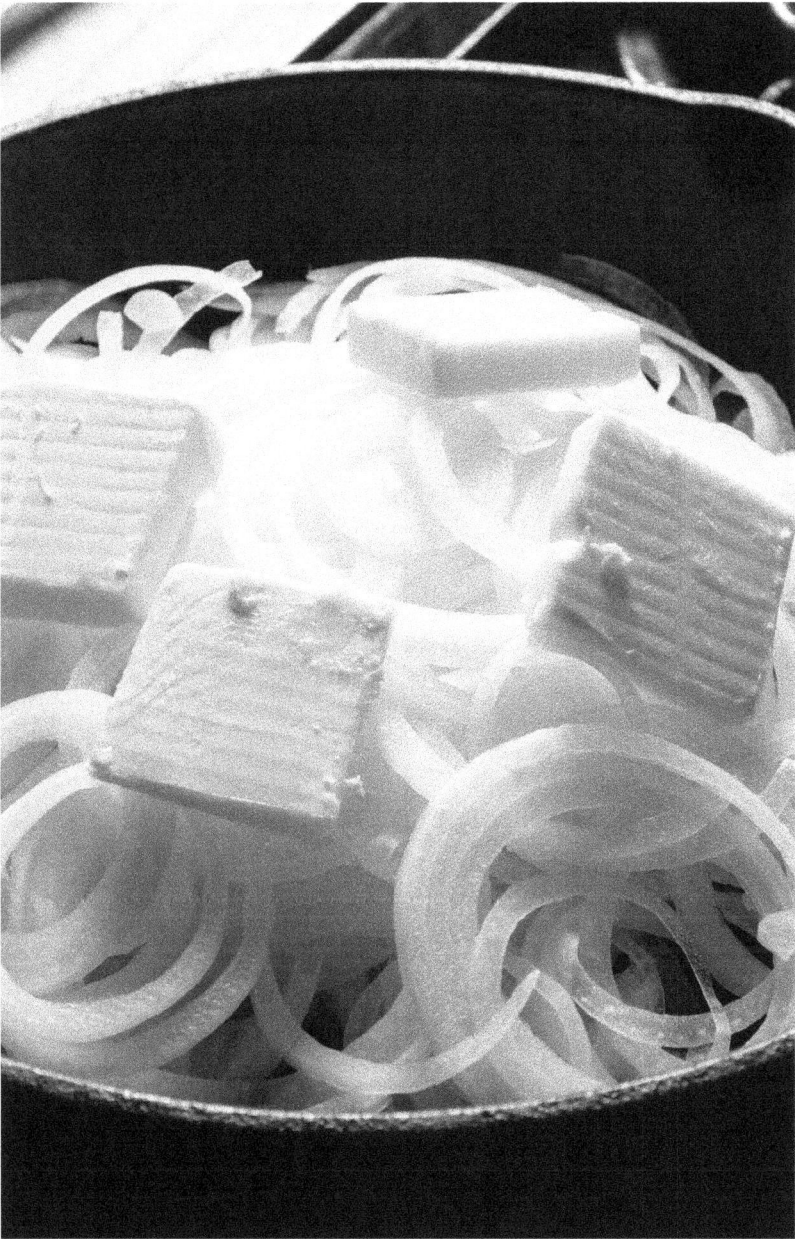

Broccoli Curry

Prep time: 10 minutes

Cook time: 15 minutes

Servings:4

Ingredients:

- 2 cups broccoli florets
- 1 tablespoon curry powder
- ½ cup of coconut milk
- 1 tablespoon coconut oil

Method:

1. Mix curry powder with coconut milk.

2. Melt the coconut oil in the skillet. Add broccoli florets and roast them for 3 minutes per side.

3. Then add coconut milk liquid and carefully mix the broccoli.

4. Close the lid and simmer the broccoli for 8 minutes on medium heat.

Nutritional info per serve: Calories 119, Fat 10.9, Fiber 2.4, Carbs 5.6, Protein 2.2

Keto Tomatoes

Prep time: 10 minutes

Cook time: 0 minutes

Servings: 2

Ingredients:

- 1 tomato, roughly sliced
- 1 teaspoon sesame oil
- ½ teaspoon sesame seeds
- ¼ teaspoon salt

Method:

1. Put the sliced tomato on the plate in one layer.

2. Then sprinkle it with sesame oil, salt, and sesame seeds.

Nutritional info per serve: Calories 30, Fat 2.7, Fiber 0.5, Carbs 1.4, Protein 0.4

Lime Green Beans

Prep time: 10 minutes

Cook time: 25 minutes

Servings:4

Ingredients:

- 2 cups green beans
- 1 teaspoon lime zest, grated
- 1 tablespoon lime juice
- 2 tablespoons coconut oil
- ¼ cup of water

Method:

1. Roast the green beans in the coconut oil for 3 minutes per side.

2. Then sprinkle the green beans with lime juice and lime zest.

3. Add water and close the lid.

4. Cook the green beans on medium heat for 15 minutes.

Nutritional info per serve: Calories 76, Fat 6.9, Fiber 1.9, Carbs 4, Protein 1

Mustard Asparagus

Prep time: 5 minutes

Cook time: 20 minutes

Servings: 4

Ingredients:

- 1-pound asparagus, roughly chopped
- 1 cup of water
- 1 tablespoon mustard
- 1 teaspoon avocado oil
- ½ teaspoon sesame oil

Method:

1. Roast asparagus in avocado oil for 5 minutes per side on low heat.

2. Then add water and boil the asparagus for 10 minutes.

3. Remove the asparagus from the water and sprinkle with sesame oil and mustard.

4. Shake the vegetables before serving.

Nutritional info per serve: Calories 42, Fat 1.7, Fiber 2.8, Carbs 5.5, Protein 3.2

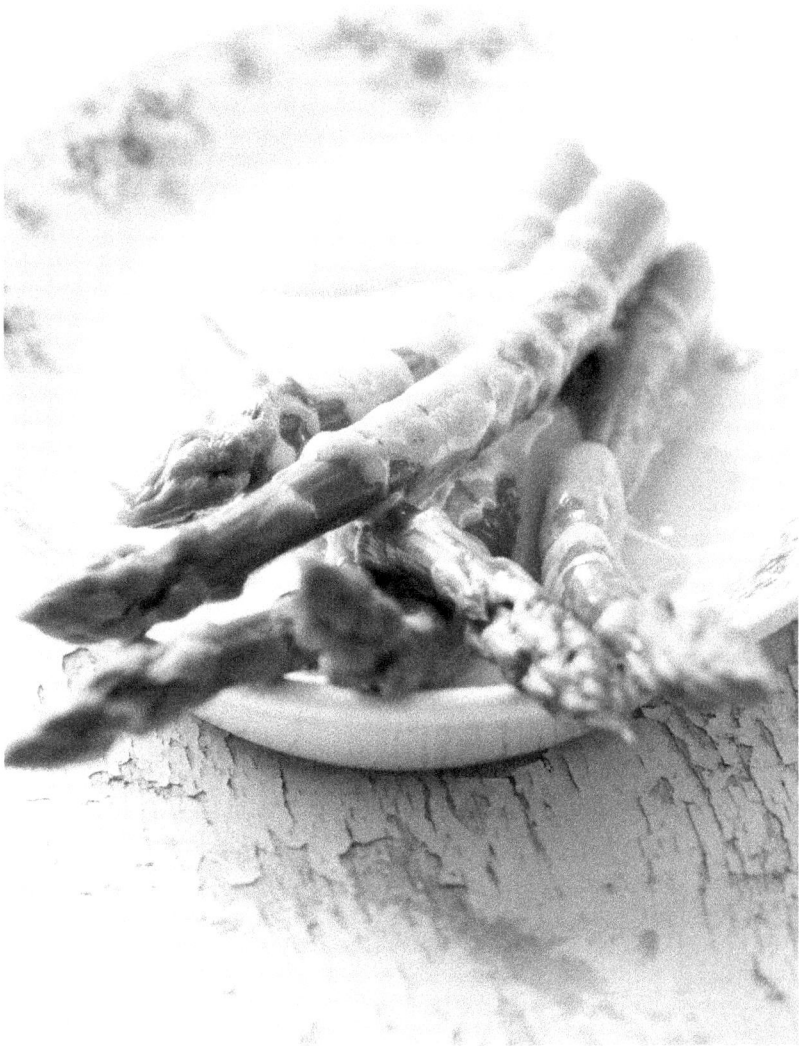

Baked Kale

Prep time: 10 minutes

Cook time: 15 minutes

Servings:6

Ingredients:

- 5 cups kale, roughly chopped
- 1 teaspoon olive oil
- 1 teaspoon smoked paprika
- 2 oz Parmesan, grated

Method:

1. Brush the baking pan with olive oil.

2. Then mix kale with smoked paprika and Parmesan.

3. Put the mixture in the baking pan and bake it for 15 minutes at 360F.

Nutritional info per serve: Calories 66, Fat 2.8, Fiber 1, Carbs 6.4, Protein 4.8

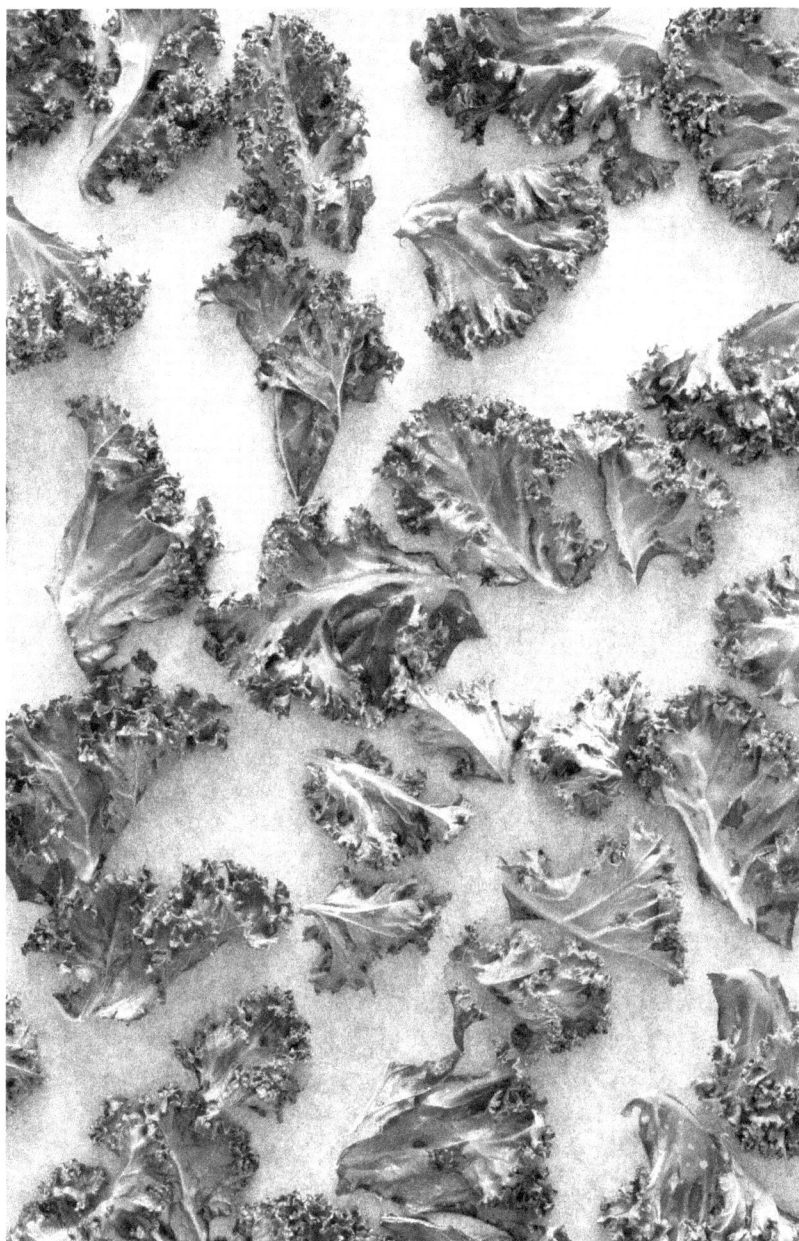

Baked Collard Greens

Prep time: 10 minutes

Cook time: 10 minutes

Servings: 4

Ingredients:

- 1 teaspoon chipotle powder
- 2 cups collard greens, chopped
- 1 tablespoon sesame oil
- 1 teaspoon ground black pepper

Method:

1. Preheat the sesame oil well.

2. Add collard greens, ground black pepper, and chipotle powder.

3. Carefully mix the greens and cook them for 10 minutes.

Nutritional info per serve: Calories 38, Fat 3.6, Fiber 0.9, Carbs 1.6, Protein 0.6

Cumin Cauliflower

Prep time: 10 minutes

Cook time: 20 minutes

Servings:6

Ingredients:

- 3 cups cauliflower florets
- 2 cups of water
- 1 teaspoon cumin seeds
- 1 tablespoon coconut oil
- ½ teaspoon ground turmeric

Method:

1. Boil the cauliflower in the water for 10 minutes.

2. Then drain water and add cumin seeds, coconut oil, and ground turmeric.

3. Shake the cauliflower gently and roast for 5 minutes.

Nutritional info per serve: Calories 34, Fat 2.4, Fiber 1.3, Carbs 2.9, Protein 1.1

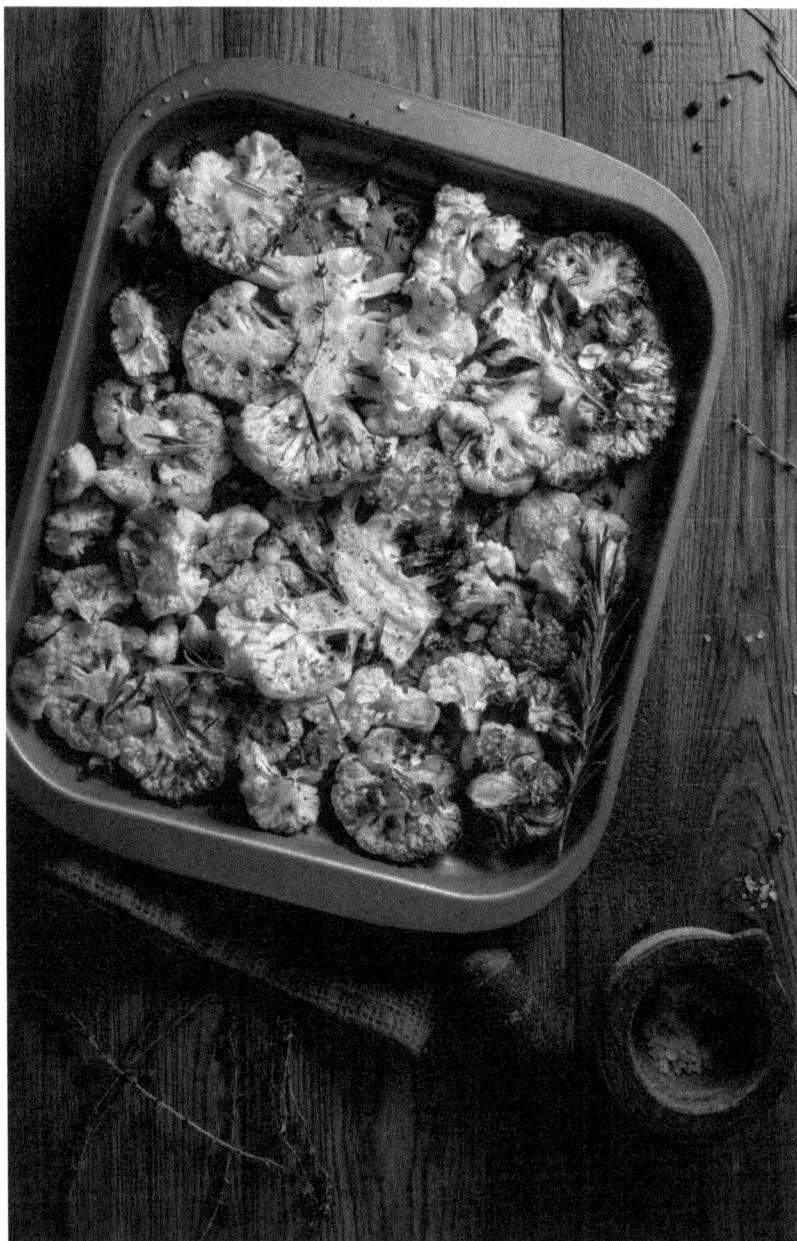

Asparagus Soup

Prep time: 10 minutes

Cook time: 20 minutes

Servings: 4

Ingredients:

- 4 cups chicken broth
- ½ cup of coconut milk
- 10 oz asparagus, chopped
- 1 teaspoon butter
- ½ carrot, diced
- 1 teaspoon dried oregano
- 1 teaspoon garlic powder

Method:

1. Put the butter in the saucepan. Melt it.

2. Add asparagus and roast it for 5 minutes.

3. Then add all remaining ingredients.

4. Simmer the soup for 15 minutes on medium heat.

Nutritional info per serve: Calories 137, Fat 9.6, Fiber 2.6, Carbs 6.8, Protein 7.3

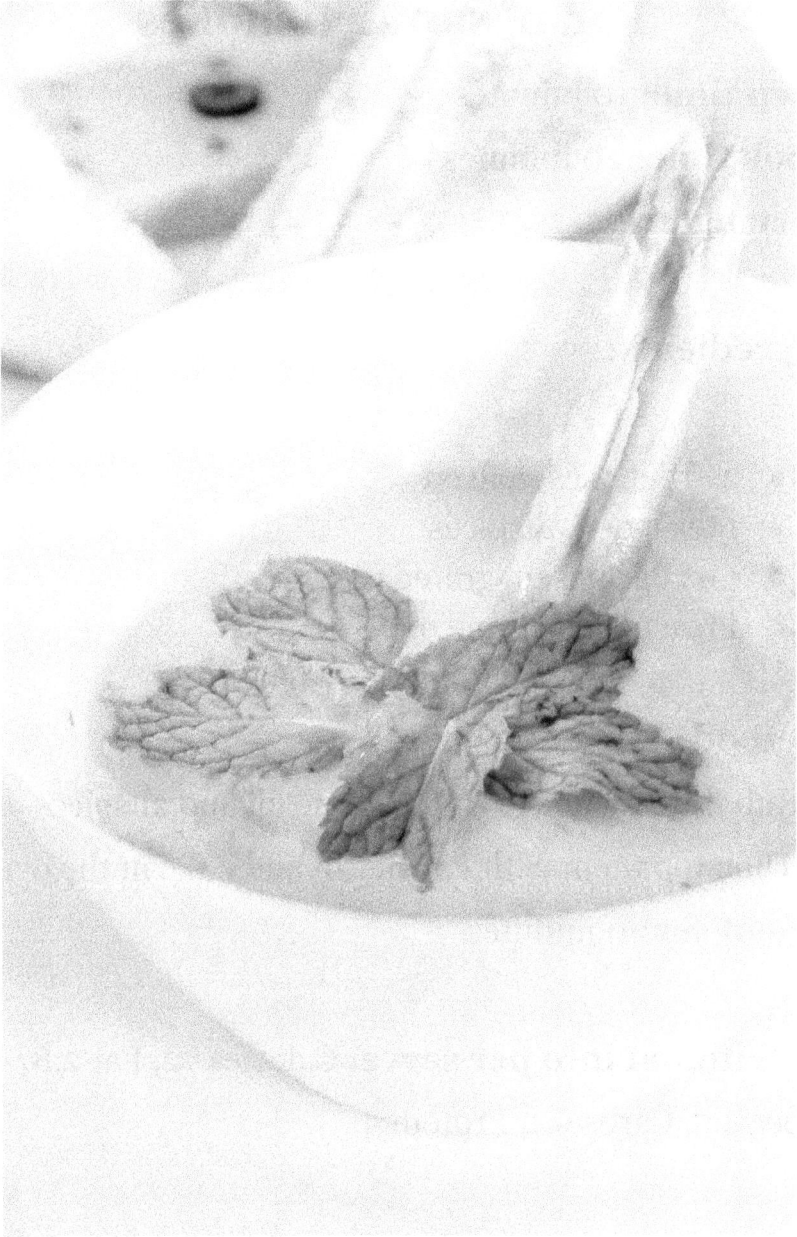

Parmesan Artichokes

Prep time: 10 minutes

Cook time: 20 minutes

Servings:4

Ingredients:

- 2 artichokes, halved
- 1 teaspoon allspices
- 1 oz Parmesan, grated
- 1 teaspoon sesame oil

Method:

1. Rub the artichokes with sesame oil and allspices.

2. Then top them with Parmesan and bake in the oven at 360F for 20 minutes.

Nutritional info per serve: Calories 72, Fat 2.8, Fiber 4.5, Carbs 9.1, Protein 5

Mustard Greens Soup

Prep time: 10 minutes

Cook time: 30 minutes

Servings: 4

Ingredients:

- 2 cups mustard greens, chopped
- 2 cups collard greens, chopped
- 3 quarts vegetable stock
- 1 onion, peeled and chopped
- Salt and ground black pepper, to taste
- 2 tablespoons coconut aminos
- 2 teaspoons fresh ginger, grated

Method:

1. Put the stock into a saucepan and bring to a simmer over medium-high heat.

2. Add mustard, collard greens, onion, salt, pepper, coconut aminos, ginger, stir, cover the pan, and cook for 30 minutes.

3. Blend the soup using an immersion blender, add more salt, and pepper, heat up over medium heat, ladle into soup bowls, and serve.

Nutritional info per serve: Calories 35, Fat 0.4, Fiber 2.8, Carbs 7, Protein 1.9

Rutabaga Cakes

Prep time: 15 minutes

Cook time: 25 minutes

Servings:4

Ingredients:

- 8 oz rutabaga, diced
- 2 eggs, beaten
- 1 teaspoon ground coriander
- 3 tablespoons almond flour
- 1 teaspoon ground paprika
- 1 tablespoon coconut oil
- ¼ cup coconut cream

Method:

1. Mix rutabaga with eggs, ground coriander, almond flour, ground paprika, and coconut cream.

2. Then grease the baking pan with coconut oil.

3. Make the small cakes from the rutabaga mixture and put them in the prepared baking pan.

4. Bake the rutabaga cakes at 365F for 25 minutes.

Nutritional info per serve: Calories 147, Fat 12, Fiber 2.5, Carbs 7, Protein 5

Greens Soup

Prep time: 5 minutes

Cook time: 20 minutes

Servings: 6

Ingredients:

- 6 cups chicken broth
- 2 cups fresh spinach, chopped
- 1 teaspoon ginger powder
- ½ cup turnip, chopped
- ½ cup coconut cream
- ½ teaspoon dried oregano
- ½ teaspoon salt

Method:

1. Put all ingredients in the saucepan and mix.

2. Close the lid and boil the soup for 20 minutes on medium-low heat.

Nutritional info per serve: Calories 91, Fat 6.2, Fiber 1, Carbs 3.4, Protein 5.7

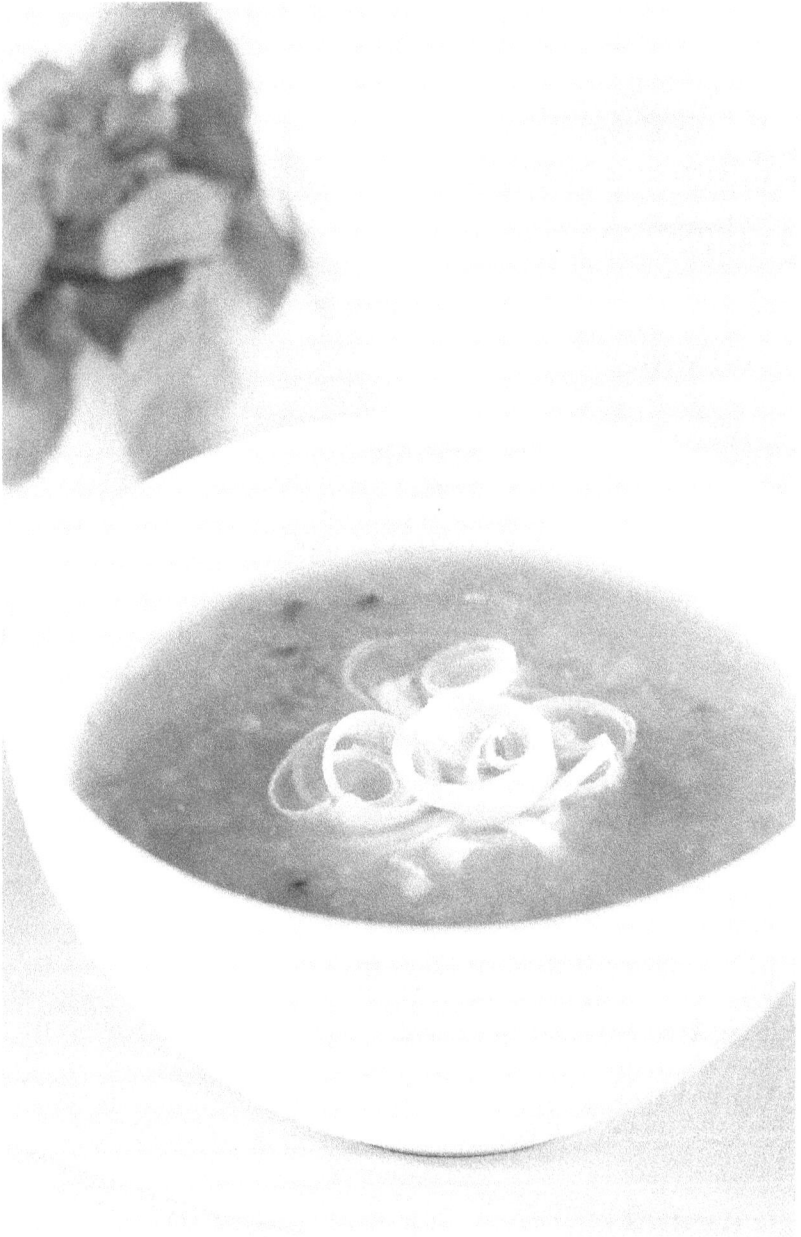

Cheese Edamame Beans

Prep time: 10 minutes

Cook time: 15 minutes

Servings:2

Ingredients:

- 1 cup edamame beans, cooked
- ¼ cup Provolone cheese, shredded
- 1 teaspoon coconut oil
- ¼ teaspoon ground black pepper
- ½ teaspoon apple cider vinegar

Method:

1. Roast the edamame beans with coconut oil for 2 minutes.

2. Then add ground black pepper and apple cider vinegar. Mix the vegetables.

3. Add Provolone cheese and close the lid.

4. Cook the meal on medium heat for 10 minutes.

Nutritional info per serve: Calories 137, Fat 7, Fiber 3.8, Carbs 11, Protein 8.2

Cilantro Asparagus

Prep time: 10 minutes

Cook time: 20 minutes

Servings: 3

Ingredients:

- 1 asparagus bunch, trimmed
- 3 teaspoons sesame oil
- 1 teaspoon apple cider vinegar
- 1 tablespoon dried oregano

Method:

1. Roast the asparagus in the sesame oil for 4 minutes per side.

2. Then add dried oregano and apple cider vinegar. Stir the asparagus.

3. Close the lid and cook it for 10 minutes on low heat.

Nutritional info per serve: Calories 54, Fat 4.7, Fiber 1.6, Carbs 2.7, Protein 1.2

Sauteed Collard Greens

Prep time: 10 minutes

Cook time: 10 minutes

Servings:2

Ingredients:

- 1 cup Collard Greens
- 1 teaspoon apple cider vinegar
- 1 teaspoon ground black pepper
- ½ cup of coconut milk

Method:

1. Pour coconut milk in the saucepan and bring it to boil.

2. Add collard greens and ground black pepper. Boil the greens for 5 minutes.

3. Then add apple cider vinegar and remove the meal from the heat.

Nutritional info per serve: Calories 147, Fat 14.5, Fiber 2.4, Carbs 5.3, Protein 2

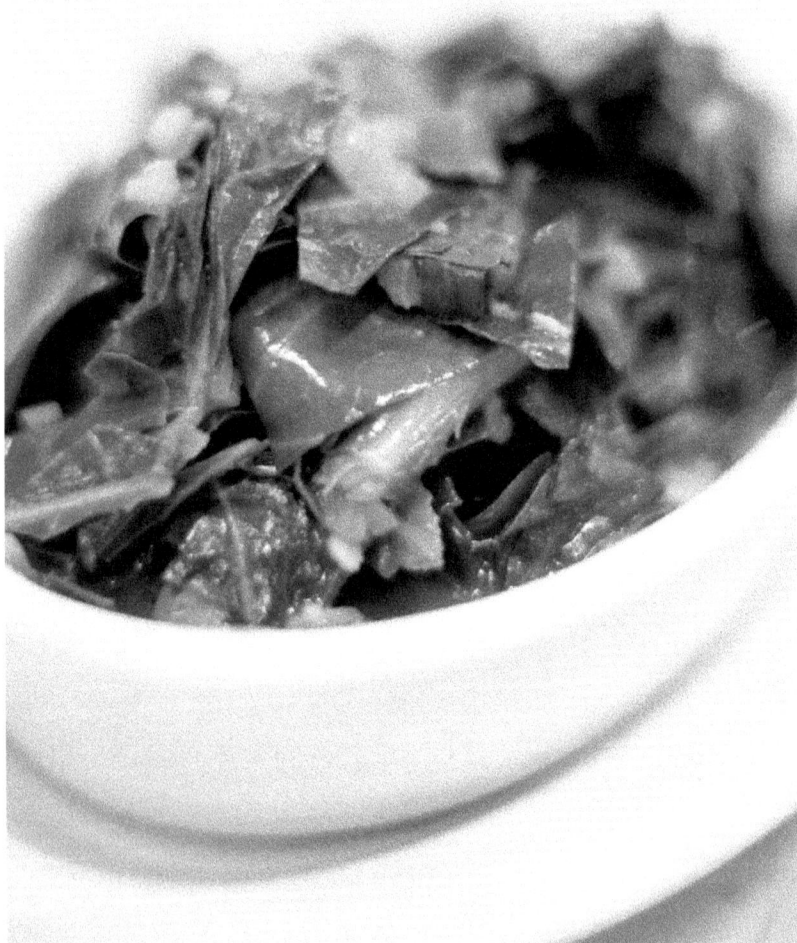

Spinach Fritters

Prep time: 10 minutes

Cook time: 10 minutes

Servings: 2

Ingredients:

- 2 cups spinach, chopped
- 2 eggs, beaten
- 2 oz Cheddar cheese, shredded
- 2 tablespoons coconut flour
- ½ teaspoon chili powder
- 1 tablespoon sesame oil

Method:

1. Mix spinach with eggs, Cheddar cheese, coconut flour, and chili powder.

2. Then preheat the sesame oil in the skillet well.

3. Make the fritters from the spinach mixture and put them in the hot oil.

4. Roast the fritters for 5 minutes per side on the medium heat.

Nutritional info per serve: Calories 281, Fat 22.1, Fiber 3.9, Carbs 6.7, Protein 15

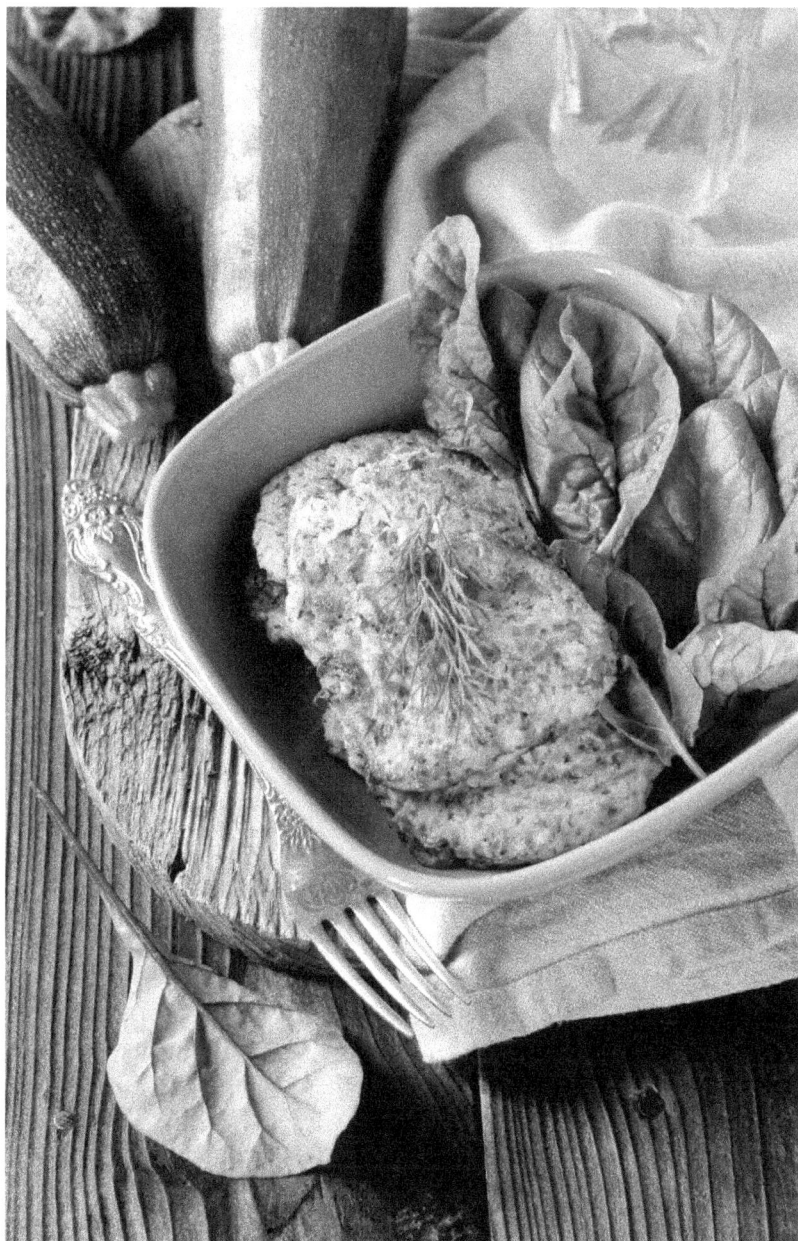

Oregano Eggplants

Prep time: 10 minutes

Cook time: 10 minutes

Servings:3

Ingredients:

- 2 eggplants, sliced
- 1 teaspoon salt
- 1 tablespoon coconut oil
- 1 tablespoon dried oregano

Method:

1. Mix the eggplants with salt and dried oregano.

2. Then melt the coconut oil in the skillet.

3. Add the eggplants. Flatten in one layer and roast them for 2 minutes per side.

Nutritional info per serve: Calories 86, Fat 7.6, Fiber 0.6, Carbs 1.2, Protein 3.9

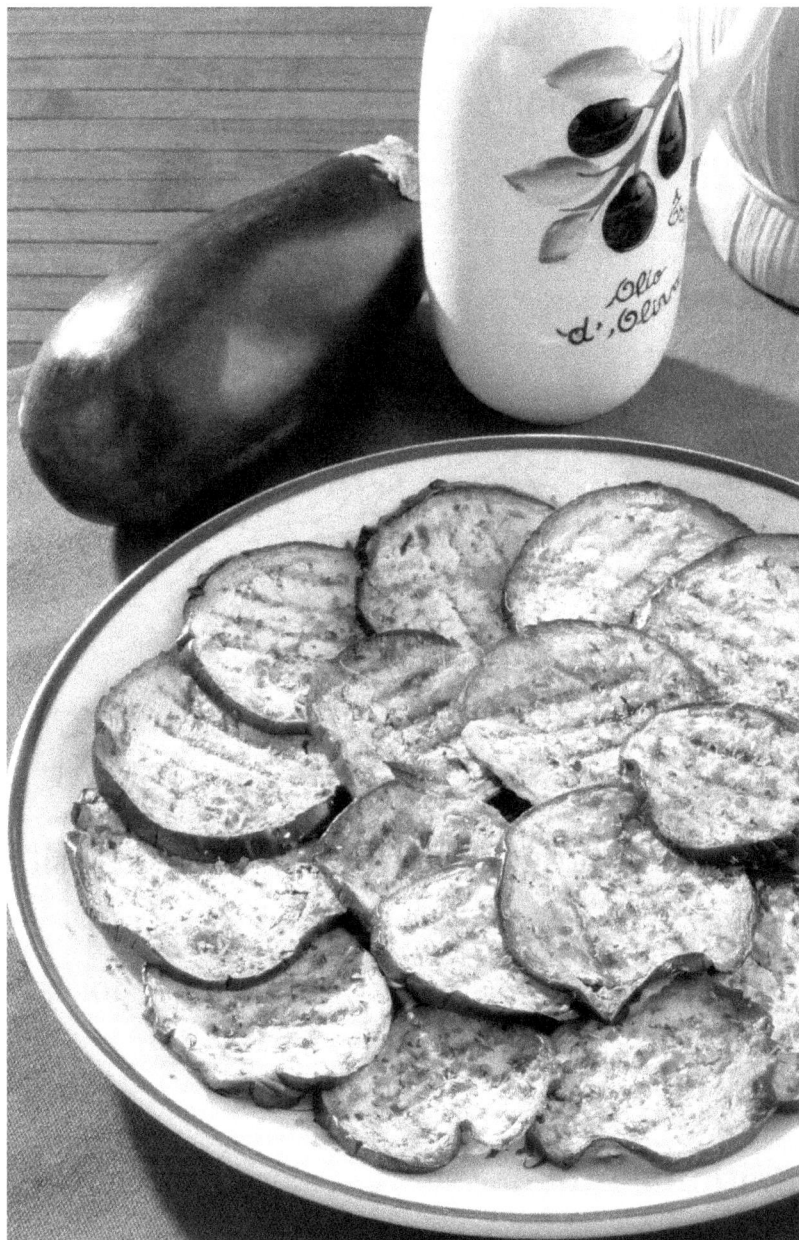

Yogurt Asparagus

Prep time: 10 minutes

Cook time: 15 minutes

Servings: 4

Ingredients:

- ½ cup Plain yogurt
- 1 teaspoon chili flakes
- 1-pound asparagus, chopped
- ½ cup of water
- ½ teaspoon salt

Method:

1. Mix plain yogurt with chili flakes, water, and salt and pour in the saucepan.

2. Add asparagus and simmer the vegetables for 15 minutes on medium high heat.

Nutritional info per serve: Calories 45, Fat 0.5, Fiber 2.4, Carbs 6.6, Protein 4.2

Avocado and Walnut Bowl

Prep time: 10 minutes

Cook time: 0 minutes

Servings:2

Ingredients:

- 1 avocado, pitted, halved, chopped
- 1 oz walnuts, chopped
- 1 oz Parmesan, chopped
- 1 teaspoon olive oil
- 1 teaspoon Italian seasonings

Method:

1. Put the avocado in the bowl.

2. Add walnuts, Parmesan, olive oil, and Italian seasonings.

3. Shake the ingredients well.

Nutritional info per serve: Calories 365, Fat 34, Fiber 7.7, Carbs 10.8, Protein 9.9

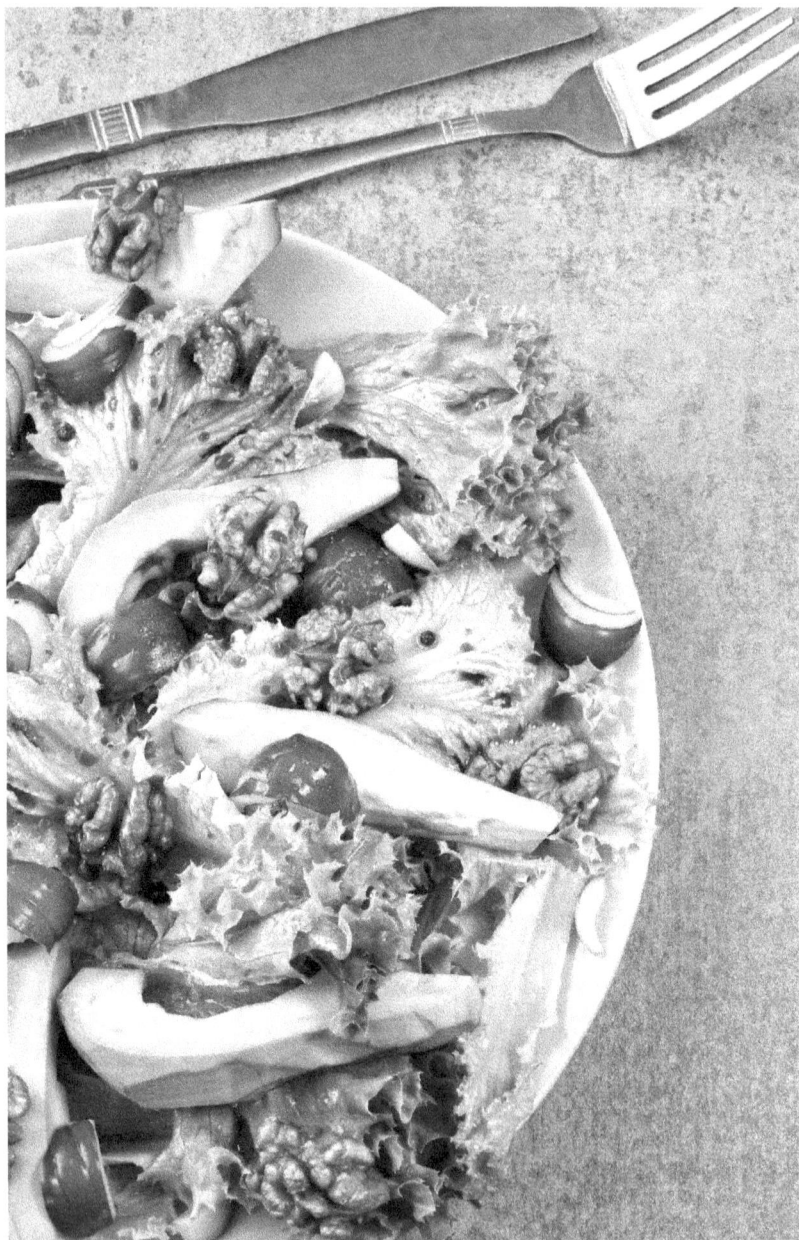

Greens Omelette

Prep time: 10 minutes

Cook time: 10 minutes

Servings: 4

Ingredients:

- ½ cup of coconut milk
- 4 eggs, beaten
- 1 cup spinach, chopped
- ¼ cup asparagus, chopped
- 1 tablespoon butter
- ½ teaspoon salt

Method:

1. Mix eggs with coconut milk and salt.

2. Then melt butter in the skillet.

3. Add egg mixture and spinach.

4. Close the lid and cook the omelet for 10 minutes on low heat.

Nutritional info per serve: Calories 161, Fat 14.4, Fiber 1, Carbs 2.6, Protein 6.7

Asparagus Masala

Prep time: 10 minutes

Cook time: 20 minutes

Servings:4

Ingredients:

- 1-pound asparagus, chopped
- 1 cup coconut cream
- 1 teaspoon butter
- 1 teaspoon garam masala

Method:

1. Melt the butter in the saucepan.

2. Add asparagus and roast it for 3 minutes per side.

3. Add garam masala and coconut cream.

4. Close the lid and cook the vegetables for 10 minutes.

Nutritional info per serve: Calories 169, Fat 15.4, Fiber 3.7, Carbs 7.7, Protein 3.9

Monterey Jack Cheese Asparagus

Prep time: 10 minutes

Cook time: 25 minutes

Servings: 3

Ingredients:

- 10 oz asparagus, chopped
- ½ cup Monterey Jack Cheese, shredded
- 1 tablespoon cream cheese
- 1 teaspoon mustard
- 1 teaspoon butter, softened
- ¼ cup of water

Method:

1. Grease the baking pan with butter and put asparagus inside.

2. Add mustard, cream cheese, and water.

3. Then add Monterey Jack cheese and bake the meal in the oven at 365F for 25 minutes.

Nutritional info per serve: Calories 117, Fat 8.6, Fiber 2.1, Carbs 4.3, Protein 7.2

Chives Fritters

Prep time: 10 minutes

Cook time: 10 minutes

Servings:2

Ingredients:

- 1 cup broccoli, shredded
- 1 tablespoon chives
- 1 egg, beaten
- 1 teaspoon ground black pepper
- 1/3 cup almond flour
- 1 tablespoon avocado oil

Method:

1. Mix broccoli with chives, egg, ground black pepper, and almond flour.

2. Preheat the avocado oil in the skillet.

3. Make the fritters from the chives mixture and roast them in hot oil for 3 minutes per side.

Nutritional info per serve: Calories 86, Fat 5.6, Fiber 2.3, Carbs 5.3, Protein 5.3

Sprouts Salad

Prep time: 10 minutes

Cook time: 0 minutes

Servings: 4

Ingredients:

- 2 cups Brussel sprouts, boiled
- 1 pecan, chopped
- 1 /4 cup plain yogurt
- 1 tablespoon fresh dill, chopped
- 1 tablespoon lemon juice

Method:

1. Mix all ingredients in a salad bowl.

2. Stir the salad.

Nutritional info per serve: Calories 57, Fat 2.9, Fiber 2.2, Carbs 6.1, Protein 2.9

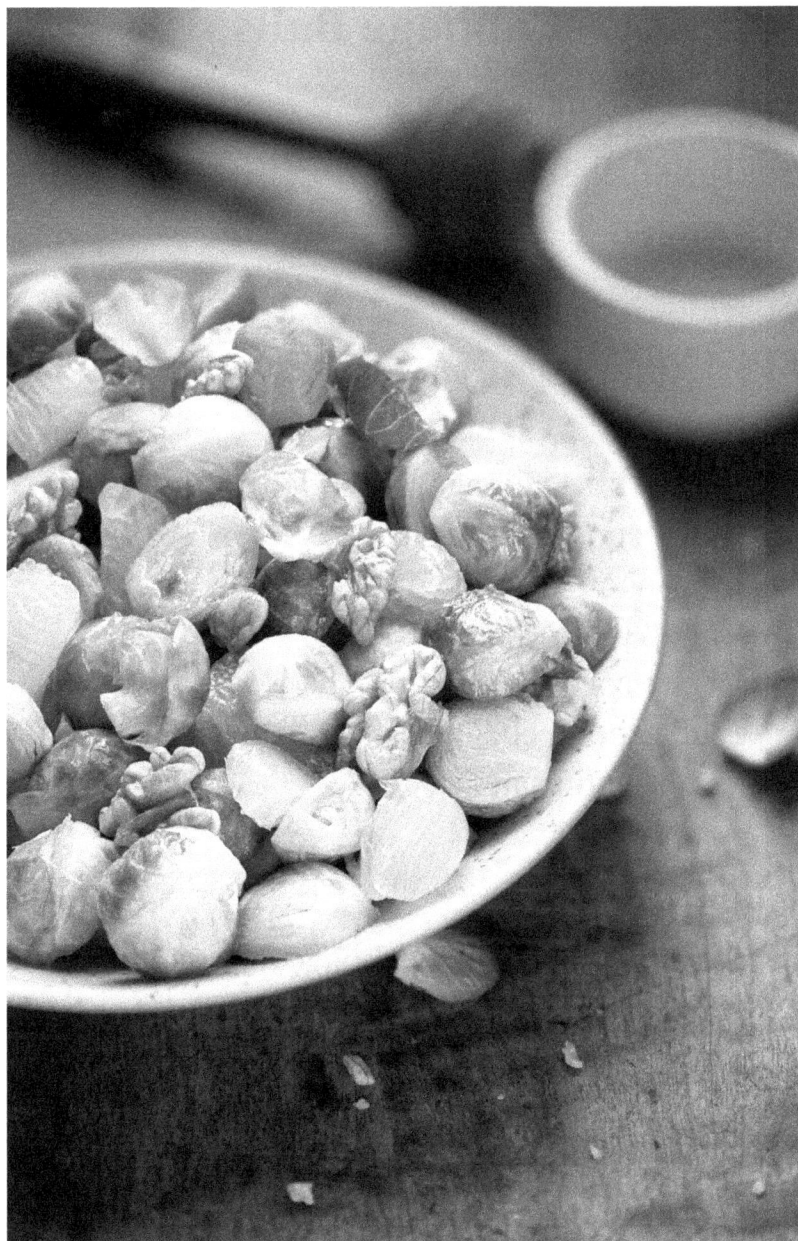

Cabbage Balls

Prep time: 10 minutes

Cook time: 10 minutes

Servings:3

Ingredients:

- 1 cup white cabbage, shredded
- 1 tablespoon hemp seeds
- 1 teaspoon ground coriander
- ¼ cup plain yogurt
- ½ cup coconut flour
- 1 tablespoon coconut oil
- ½ teaspoon salt

Method:

1. In the mixing bowl, mix cabbage, hemp seeds, ground coriander, yogurt, coconut flour, and salt.

2. Make the balls from the cabbage mixture and put them in the hot skillet.

3. Add coconut oil and roast the cabbage balls for 4 minutes per side or until they are golden brown.

Nutritional info per serve: Calories 71, Fat 5.2, Fiber 1.6, Carbs 4.4, Protein 1.9

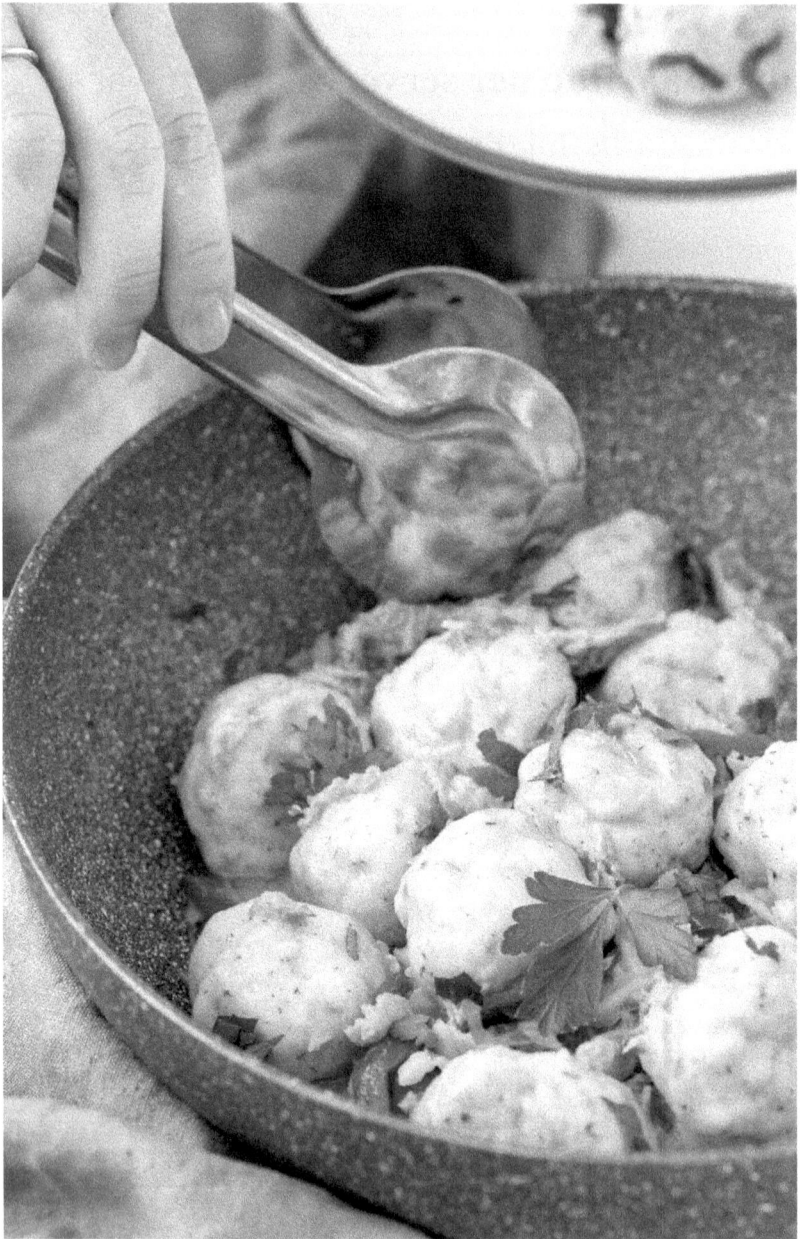

Turmeric Radishes

Prep time: 10 minutes

Cook time: 15 minutes

Servings: 2

Ingredients:

- 2 cups radishes, halved
- 2 tablespoons coconut oil
- 1 teaspoon ground turmeric
- 1 teaspoon salt

Method:

1. Mix the radishes with coconut oil, ground turmeric, and salt.

2. Put the mixture in the baking tray and roast it for 15 minutes in the oven at 365F.

Nutritional info per serve: Calories 140, Fat 13.8, Fiber 2.1, Carbs 4.7, Protein 0.9

Jicama Noodles

Prep time: 15 minutes

Cook time: 8 minutes

Servings:6

Ingredients:

- 1-pound jicama, peeled
- 2 tablespoons coconut cream
- 1 teaspoon sesame oil
- ½ teaspoon dried cilantro

Method:

1. Spiralize the jicama with the help of the spiralizer.

2. Then preheat the sesame oil in the skillet.

3. Add jicama noodles, dried cilantro, and coconut cream.

4. Stir the mixture and cook it on medium heat for 5 minutes.

Nutritional info per serve: Calories 47, Fat 2, Fiber 3.8, Carbs 7, Protein 0.7

Rosemary Radish

Prep time: 10 minutes

Cook time: 10 minutes

Servings: 4

Ingredients:

- 1-pound radish, sliced
- 1 teaspoon dried rosemary
- 1 tablespoon butter

Method:

1. Melt the butter in the skillet.

2. Then add radish and dried rosemary.

3. Roast the radish for 10 minutes. Stir the meal from time to time.

Nutritional info per serve: Calories 45, Fat 3, Fiber 1.9, Carbs 4.1, Protein 0.8

Broccoli Slaw

Prep time: 15 minutes

Cook time: 5 minutes

Servings:4

Ingredients:

- 1 cup broccoli, shredded
- 1 tablespoon plain yogurt
- 1 teaspoon sesame oil
- 1 teaspoon sesame seeds
- 1 tablespoon lime juice
- 1 teaspoon butter
- 1 cup white cabbage, shredded

Method:

1. Roast the shredded broccoli with butter for 5 minutes. Stir it from time to time.

2. Then mix cooked broccoli with plain yogurt, sesame oil, sesame seeds, lime juice, and white cabbage.

3. Carefully mix the meal.

Nutritional info per serve: Calories 39, Fat 2.6, Fiber 1.2, Carbs 3.5, Protein 1.2

Coated Radish

Prep time: 10 minutes

Cook time: 10 minutes

Servings: 4

Ingredients:

- 2 eggs, beaten
- 1 cup radish, trimmed
- 1 tablespoon coconut oil
- 3 tablespoons coconut flour

Method:

1. Dip the radish in the eggs and then coat in the coconut flour.

2. Preheat the coconut oil well.

3. Add the coated radishes in the hot coconut oil and roast for 2-3 minutes or until radishes are golden brown.

Nutritional info per serve: Calories 88, Fat 6.4, Fiber 2.3, Carbs 4.2, Protein 3.7

www.ingramcontent.com/pod-product-compliance
Lightning Source LLC
Chambersburg PA
CBHW050757030426
42336CB00012B/1863